Root & Recalibrate

Clearing the Gut, Lymph & Spirit for Sustainable Balance

Volume I
The Rooted Body Series

Zaire Sabb, PhD(C)

text is expressly prohibited. The author reserves all rights to license uses of this work for generative AI training and development of machine learning language models.
This book may not be used for commercial purposes, trainings, or distributed in whole or in part without express written permission.

First Edition
ISBN: 979-8-9990186-4-9

Cover design by: Harry Lawson (Enigma Graphics)
Editing & Interior layout by: Chelsia McCoy/*Your Writing Table*)
(www.yourwritingtable.com)

Published by Sacred Roots Press
An imprint of Earth & Ink Publishing, LLC
Printed in United States of America.

Table of Contents

Introduction

The Purpose of this reset...

In every cycle of growth, there comes a time to pause, purge, and prepare the soil for what's next. *Root & Recalibrate* was born out of that sacred necessity. The need to return to the foundation, clear what no longer serves and align the body, mind, and spirit with purpose. This 21-day reset is not a trend or a quick fix. It is a ritual of remembrance and reclamation.

Over a decade ago, I created this reset to support my own healing—physically, spiritually, and energetically. What started as a personal recalibration became a guiding protocol I've offered to clients and community with transformative results. While the outer world pushes constant consumption, this reset invites you into conscious release. It is a call to simplify, to slow down, to listen to your body's messages, and to honor your spiritual integrity.

This work is rooted in ancestral wisdom, informed by clinical experience, and shaped by years of supporting people through the sacred process of detoxification. Here, the gut is not just a physical place, but a spiritual gateway. When the gut is stagnated, so is the spirit. When the digestive fire dims, clarity, vitality, and direction fade. Reigniting that fire is the first step toward remembering who you are beyond the toxins, the trauma, and the tension.

"Recalibration of the self" is the heart of this offering. Through dietary shifts, herbal ally incorporation, spiritual rituals, and ancestral practices, this guide provides a path back to your center.

Whether you are cleansing for the first time or returning for a seasonal reset, know this: every time you choose to align, you choose life. You choose legacy. You choose liberation.

Understanding the 21-Day Reset

The *21-Day Reset* is a sacred container for intentional cleansing and spiritual discipline. It is a holistic approach that touches every layer of the self—physical, emotional, energetic, and ancestral. Rooted in African healing traditions, spiritual hygiene, and functional wellness, this reset is structured to help you pause, purge, and realign.

Unlike many detox programs that focus solely on food, this reset honors the truth that wellness is multidimensional. The body cannot fully detox if the mind is heavy. The spirit cannot soar if the gut is stagnated. Through specific abstentions, daily rituals, herbal supports, and conscious nourishment, this protocol invites you into a space of clarity, softness, and spiritual fortification.

The Core Principles

- **Discipline as Devotion**: Every "no" in this protocol is a "yes" to something deeper. By abstaining from meat, dairy, processed sugars, sexual activity, and other stimulants, you give your body and spirit space to recalibrate.
- **Spiritual Cleanliness**: Wearing all white is not just aesthetic, it's energetic. This practice, along

with daily bathing rituals, prayer, and meditation, creates a protective and clarifying spiritual field.

- **Daily Rhythm**: From sunrise prayer to nightly ancestor meditation, the reset creates a rhythm that connects you to natural cycles. Ritual bathing with black soap and a loofah supports physical and energetic shedding.
- **Herbal and Nutritional Support**: A plant-based diet rich in fruits, vegetables, grains, and hydration supports detox pathways. The optional herbal protocols (for parasites, lymph, and gut health) deepen the physical cleanse.
- **Colon Hydrotherapy or Oral Colonics**: Three sessions, at the beginning, middle, and end, help flush physical waste and energetic residue. Alternatives are provided for those unable to access hydrotherapy.

Why 21 Days?

In traditional healing and spiritual disciplines, 21 days is considered a full cycle of transformation. It allows the body to release old patterns and begin new ones, while giving the spirit time to catch up. Three weeks is long enough to be challenging, but short enough to remain focused and intentional. The chapters that follow will guide you through the physiological, emotional, and spiritual dimensions of this recalibration.

Why the Gut Is the Root

- Anatomy and physiology of digestion
- Gut stagnation and systemic inflammation
- Interconnection with skin, respiratory, cardiovascular, immune, and neurological systems
- Gut-brain axis and mood regulation
- Gut-liver axis and detox pathways

The gut is more than a digestive system it is the core of our physical health, our emotional well-being, and our spiritual clarity. Known in many traditions as the "second brain," the gut is where nourishment becomes vitality or stagnation becomes imbalance. When the gut is out of alignment, the entire body suffers. When it is functioning well, it becomes a sacred root from which all other systems can thrive.

In clinical terms, the gut houses a vast and intelligent ecosystem known as the microbiome, a diverse population of bacteria that play key roles in digestion, detoxification, immunity, hormone balance, and mood regulation. In spiritual terms, it is a seat of intuition, where we feel truth in our bellies, where ancestral wisdom can land, and where unresolved emotional residue is often stored.

Stagnation Spreads

When digestion slows or becomes impaired (through poor eating habits, stress, toxins, or lack of movement) it causes gut stagnation, leading to:

- Bloating, gas, and constipation
- Toxin buildup in the bloodstream
- Inflammation that affects joints, skin, and the brain
- Overgrowth of parasites or candida
- Disrupted immune responses

This stagnation doesn't stay in the gut; it spreads outward, weakening the body's systems and dulling the clarity of the spirit. It becomes harder to focus, harder to sleep, harder to hear your own internal guidance. The fog isn't just in the mind; it's coming from the gut.

Interconnected Body Systems

Here's how gut dysfunction shows up in other areas:

- **Skin**: Acne, rashes, eczema, and chronic breakouts often indicate liver overload or gut imbalance.
- **Immune System**: 70% of immune cells live in the gut. Dysbiosis (microbial imbalance) can cause autoimmune flare-ups, food sensitivities, and chronic fatigue.

- **Nervous System**: Gut stagnation can lead to anxiety, depression, irritability, and poor stress response due to the gut-brain axis.
- **Liver & Detox Pathways**: A sluggish gut burdens the liver, preventing efficient removal of toxins and estrogens from the body.
- **Lymphatic System:** When waste isn't properly eliminated through the colon, the lymph system becomes congested, leading to swelling, inflammation, and low vitality.

  Over time, chronic lymphatic congestion allows inflammatory mediators, toxins, and can potentially assist malignant or pre-malignant cells to circulate rather than be neutralized and cleared. This impaired immune surveillance and fluid stagnation is one of the primary mechanisms through which metastasis occurs, as abnormal cells migrate through lymphatic channels to distant tissues instead of being contained and eliminated.

Reproductive Manifestations of Gut Stagnation

Because the digestive system plays a central role in hormone metabolism, immune regulation, and inflammatory control, gut stagnation often expresses itself through the reproductive system. This occurs in sex-specific ways, though the underlying mechanisms such as impaired detoxification, altered microbiota, and chronic inflammation are shared.

In the Female Reproductive System

Gut stagnation may contribute to:

- **Estrogen recirculation and hormonal congestion**

  Slowed bowel transit and dysbiosis impair estrogen clearance via the estrobolome, increasing circulating estrogen. The estrobolome refers to the collection of gut bacteria and their genes involved in estrogen metabolism. These microbes produce enzymes such as beta glucuronidase that regulate the deconjugation and recirculation of estrogens within the body. When bowel transit is slowed or the gut microbiome becomes imbalanced, estrogen clearance is impaired, resulting in increased reabsorption and elevated circulating estrogen levels, which may clinically present as fibroids, endometriosis, breast tenderness, heavy or painful menses, and cyclical mood disturbances.

  Conversely, significant alterations in microbial composition may reduce estrogen reactivation, leading to lower circulating estrogen levels. Either direction of imbalance disrupts endocrine signaling and may contribute to the development of obesity, metabolic syndrome, estrogen sensitive cancers including breast, endometrial, and ovarian cancers, endometrial hyperplasia, endometriosis, polycystic ovary syndrome, impaired fertility, cardiovascular disease, and changes in cognitive function.

- **Pelvic and uterine stagnation**
Inflammatory metabolites and lymphatic congestion originating in the gut can affect pelvic circulation, contributing to pelvic congestion, dysmenorrhea, and reproductive organ sensitivity.
- **Altered vaginal and uterine microbiota**
Disruption of gut microbial balance can influence the urogenital microbiome, increasing susceptibility to recurrent infections, inflammation, or altered cervical and vaginal environments.

In the Male Reproductive System

Gut stagnation may contribute to:

- **Testosterone suppression and estrogen dominance**
Chronic inflammation and impaired detoxification increase aromatase activity, converting testosterone into estrogen. This may present as reduced libido, erectile dysfunction, fatigue, gynecomastia, or mood instability.
- **Prostatic and pelvic inflammation**
Toxic burden and immune dysregulation originating in the gut may contribute to prostate irritation, urinary symptoms, or chronic pelvic discomfort.
- **Reduced sperm quality and fertility potential**
Oxidative stress, nutrient malabsorption, and inflammatory signaling associated with gut dysfunction can negatively impact sperm count, motility, and morphology.

In both sexes, reproductive symptoms linked to gut stagnation often coexist with fatigue, brain fog, emotional irritability, and diminished vitality. These presentations reflect not isolated organ dysfunction, but systemic imbalance where impaired digestion disrupts endocrine signaling, immune regulation, and circulatory flow.

In this way, reproductive health becomes a visible indicator of digestive and metabolic integrity. When stagnation is cleared at the gut level, reproductive systems often regain rhythm, responsiveness, and resilience.

A Sacred Center

From a spiritual lens, the gut functions as the womb of the body, even for those without a physical uterus. It is the internal chamber where nourishment is received, broken down, and transformed into vitality, intuition, and embodied knowing. Just as the womb determines what is carried, nurtured, or released, the gut governs discernment, deciding what is assimilated and what must be let go on physical, emotional, and energetic levels.

Across spiritual and ancestral traditions, the state of the gut has long been understood as central to clarity of mind and spirit. Practices such as fasting, cleansing, and bowel rituals are not merely acts of physical purification, but intentional methods of refining perception and restoring internal order. When the gut is congested or stagnant, discernment becomes clouded, intuition dulls, and the body struggles to distinguish nourishment from burden. Conversely, when the digestive center is clear and responsive, the individual experiences greater mental clarity, emotional steadiness, and spiritual receptivity.

As a result, tending to the gut is an act of sacred stewardship. Cleansing the vessel is not about punishment or deprivation, but about creating the internal conditions necessary for insight, alignment, and conscious creation to arise. The clarity of the soul is supported by the integrity of the body that houses it, and the gut stands at the threshold where matter becomes meaning.

When we begin our healing with the gut, we are not only improving digestion, we are reestablishing our relationship to ourselves and the divine.

Zaire Sabb, PhD(C)

Emotional Physiology & Organ Memory: A Traditional Chinese Medicine Perspective

While modern physiology explains how gut stagnation disrupts immunity, hormones, and neurological signaling, it does not fully account for *why* certain patterns reoccur or why emotional states so often mirror organ dysfunction. For this, we turn to traditional systems of medicine that have long recognized the body as both biological and emotional terrain. Traditional Chinese Medicine offers a framework for understanding how emotions are not merely psychological experiences, but physiological forces that influence digestion, circulation, detoxification, and disease progression. By examining the emotional body through an organ-based lens, we gain deeper insight into how unresolved emotional patterns contribute to stagnation and how true recalibration must address both the material and immaterial body.

Emotional Patterns, Organ Stagnation, and the Body's Flow

When studying healing traditions, the body has never been understood as separate from emotion. Modern research now confirms what ancestral systems have long taught: emotional states exert measurable effects on digestion, detoxification, immune function, and hormonal balance. Traditional Chinese Medicine (TCM) offers a particularly useful framework for understanding how unprocessed emotions contribute to physiological stagnation, not as metaphor, but as patterned disruption of flow.

In TCM, health is defined by the smooth movement of energy, blood, and fluids throughout the body. When this movement becomes constrained, stagnation arises. While physical factors such as diet, toxins, and inactivity certainly contribute to stagnation, emotional suppression is considered one of its most potent and underestimated causes. Emotions that are repeatedly held, inhibited, or unexpressed do not simply dissipate. They embed themselves in the body, altering organ function and impairing communication between systems.

The Liver and the Burden of Anger

Within this framework, the liver is the organ most closely associated with the emotion of anger, including its subtler expressions such as frustration, resentment, irritability, and a chronic sense of being constrained or overwhelmed. The liver governs the smooth flow of bile, blood, and metabolic waste, making it central to detoxification, digestion, and hormonal regulation.

When anger is suppressed or prolonged, liver function becomes constrained. This constraint mirrors what is clinically observed in liver stagnation: sluggish bile flow, impaired detoxification, hormonal recirculation, headaches, digestive discomfort, and a sensation of internal pressure or tension. Over time, this stagnation may contribute to estrogen dominance, menstrual irregularities, fibroids, mood volatility, and systemic inflammation.

From a Western perspective, chronic stress and emotional suppression activate the hypothalamic–pituitary–adrenal axis, increasing cortisol output and inflammatory signaling while impairing liver enzyme efficiency. Seen through both lenses, emotional tension becomes physiological burden. The liver, tasked with filtering and releasing what no longer serves, cannot perform its role fully when emotional load is left unprocessed.

The Spleen, Digestion and Emotional Overwhelm

TCM associates the spleen with digestion, assimilation, and the emotion of worry or overthinking. While Western medicine does not identify the spleen as a digestive organ in the same way, the conceptual overlap is clear. Chronic mental rumination, anxiety, and emotional overwhelm impairs appetite, digestive secretions, and gut motility, leading to bloating, fatigue, loose stools, constipation, and nutrient malabsorption.

When the digestive system is burdened by constant mental strain, the body struggles to extract nourishment efficiently. This leads to a state of depletion that further weakens detoxification pathways, immune resilience, and nervous system regulation. The cycle becomes self-perpetuating: emotional overwhelm disrupts digestion, poor digestion worsens emotional resilience, and stagnation deepens across systems.

The Lungs, Grief and the Capacity to Release

The lungs are associated in TCM with grief, loss, and the capacity to let go. They govern respiration, immune defense, and the elimination of waste through breath and skin. Prolonged grief or unresolved sorrow can manifest as shallow breathing, chronic respiratory issues, weakened immunity, and skin conditions, all of which reflect impaired elimination.

Breath serves as a primary regulator of the nervous system. When emotional pain constricts breathing patterns, oxygen delivery decreases, lymphatic movement slows, and detoxification through the lungs becomes less efficient. This reinforces the importance of breathwork and intentional respiration during periods of cleansing and recalibration.

Emotional Residue

From both a clinical and energetic standpoint, unprocessed emotions behave much like metabolic waste. They accumulate, circulate improperly, and interfere with normal physiological flow. Over time, emotional residue contributes to gut stagnation, lymphatic congestion, hormonal imbalance, and diminished vitality.

During detoxification and reset processes, it is common for emotions to surface unexpectedly. This is not regression, but release. As the body clears physical waste and improves circulation, stored emotional patterns may rise into awareness. Recognizing this process as part of healing rather than disruption allows individuals to respond with compassion rather than resistance.

Integrating Emotional Clearing into Recalibration

Recalibration requires more than dietary change or herbal support alone. It calls for awareness of the emotional patterns that contribute to immobility and intentional practices that restore flow. Breathwork, journaling, prayer, ritual bathing, and periods of stillness support the nervous system in processing emotional load while the liver, gut, and lymphatic systems resume their clearing functions.

By addressing emotional patterns alongside physical detoxification, the body is given the conditions it needs to restore coherence across systems. Flow returns not only to digestion and elimination, but to perception, clarity, and embodied presence. Considering this, emotional awareness becomes an essential component of sustainable healing, allowing recalibration to occur at the level of the whole being.

The Gut-Endocrine Connection

- The gut's role in hormone metabolism
- Dysbiosis and endocrine disruption
- The estrobolome and breast tissue health (with synthesis from PMC study)
- How gut imbalance impacts male hormone health (testosterone, prostate, fertility, mood)

The endocrine system is our body's internal messenger sending signals via hormones to regulate everything from metabolism and reproductive function to mood, energy, and immune health. But these messengers don't operate in isolation. They are deeply affected by the health of the gut.

When the gut is stagnant, inflamed, or imbalanced, it sends the wrong signals, blocks detoxification, and disrupts the flow of hormonal communication. Over time, this leads to a cascade of dysfunctions many of which show up as reproductive issues, thyroid imbalances, blood sugar instability, and even emotional volatility.

The Microbiome's Hormonal Role

The gut microbiota is involved in the modulation, metabolism, and clearance of hormones, especially estrogens and cortisol. This ecosystem breaks down excess hormones and supports the liver in processing them for safe elimination. When the gut is backed up or dysbiotic, hormones recirculate, it increases the risk of:

- Fibroids and cysts
- Irregular menstrual cycles
- Breast tenderness and density
- PMS, mood swings, and fatigue
- Estrogen-dominant conditions
- Prostatic inflammation and enlargement

In a 2020 study published in *Cancers (Basel)*, researchers confirmed that an imbalanced gut microbiome contributes to estrogen accumulation, particularly affecting breast tissue and increasing the risk for hormone-related cancers. This speaks not only to the physical risks but to the spiritual importance of digestive integrity when we cannot eliminate properly, we are forced to carry what no longer serves us.

Male Hormonal Health

Gut health also significantly impacts male hormonal balance, particularly testosterone levels and prostate health. Dysbiosis and chronic inflammation can lead to increased aromatase activity, an enzyme that converts testosterone into estrogen. This can result in:

- Decreased libido and vitality
- Mood disturbances and anxiety
- Muscle loss and increased fat retention
- Enlarged prostate or inflammation

Poor digestive hygiene, overconsumption of processed foods, and high toxin load disrupt the gut barrier, increasing systemic inflammation and reducing the body's ability to regulate and detox hormones effectively. In short: *a man's gut is deeply tied to his clarity, virility, and longevity.*

Gut Health, Libido and Vanity in Men

Libido is not just about sexual desire; it is an indicator of overall vitality, drive, and life force energy. In many traditional systems, a strong libido is a sign that the blood is circulating well, the spirit is animated, and the inner fire (sometimes called *ase*, *kundalini*, or *chi*) is flowing freely. When the gut is compromised, this fire dims.

Here's how poor gut health chips away at male libido and vitality:

- **Chronic Inflammation and Hormonal Imbalance:**
  Gut-derived inflammation increases systemic inflammatory burden, placing sustained stress on the adrenal and endocrine systems and contributing to reduced testosterone production. Simultaneously, impaired detoxification and inflammatory signaling increase aromatase activity, promoting the conversion of testosterone into estrogen, which may present clinically as reduced libido, erectile dysfunction, fatigue, gynecomastia, and mood instability.
- **Micronutrient Deficiency and Metabolic–Reproductive Disruption:**
  Gut stagnation and mucosal damage impair the absorption of critical micronutrients including zinc, magnesium, B vitamins, and essential fatty acids that are foundational for testosterone synthesis, spermatogenesis, and endocrine signaling. Over time, these deficiencies contribute to broader metabolic and reproductive disruption, manifesting as increased visceral adiposity, insulin resistance, diminished sperm quality, and reduced fertility potential.

- **Estrogen Recirculation and Prostatic Impact:** When gut elimination and microbial balance are compromised, estrogens are inadequately cleared and instead recirculate within the body, leading to estrogen overload. This hormonal imbalance contributes to fatigue, decreased libido, erectile dysfunction, and emotional instability, while also promoting prostatic inflammation and enlargement through sustained inflammatory and endocrine signaling.
- **Mood & Mental Clarity:** The gut produces over 90% of the body's serotonin, a key neurotransmitter involved in emotional regulation, sleep–wake cycles, impulse control, and motivation. Disruption of gut integrity and microbial balance impairs serotonin synthesis and signaling, often manifesting as anxiety, low mood, brain fog, diminished focus, and a reduced capacity for sexual desire, creativity, and sustained engagement with life.

Female Reproductive & Endocrine Manifestations of Gut Stagnation

In females, gut dysbiosis and impaired elimination disrupt hormonal metabolism, inflammatory balance, and pelvic circulation, often manifesting as the following interconnected patterns:

- **Estrogen Recirculation and Hormonal Congestion:**
Gut stagnation and microbial imbalance impair estrogen clearance via the estrobolome, leading to recirculation and accumulation of circulating estrogens. This hormonal congestion contributes to fibroids, ovarian cysts, breast tenderness or density, heavy or painful menses, and estrogen-dominant symptom patterns.

- **Pelvic and Uterine Stagnation:**
Chronic intestinal congestion and lymphatic overload compromise pelvic circulation and lymphatic drainage, contributing to uterine heaviness, pelvic pain, dysmenorrhea, endometriosis, and sensations of fullness or pressure within the reproductive organs.

- **Immune Dysregulation and Inflammatory Signaling:**
Increased intestinal permeability and microbial imbalance activate systemic immune responses, which may manifest as chronic pelvic inflammation, autoimmune reproductive conditions, recurrent infections, or heightened inflammatory responses during the menstrual cycle.

- **Neuroendocrine and Emotional Dysregulation:**
Disruption of gut-derived neurotransmitters (particularly serotonin) alters hypothalamic–pituitary–ovarian (HPO) axis signaling, contributing to mood instability, anxiety, irritability, sleep disturbance, premenstrual dysphoria, and diminished emotional resilience.

- **Fertility and Cyclical Rhythm Disruption:** Nutrient malabsorption, hormonal recirculation, and inflammatory burden interfere with ovulatory signaling, luteal phase integrity, and uterine receptivity, potentially contributing to irregular cycles, anovulation, implantation challenges, and reduced fertility potential.

From both a physiological and spiritual perspective, gut stagnation represents a state of diminished flow in which energy, hormones, nutrients, and purpose no longer move freely. In men, this often manifests as fatigue, loss of vitality, emotional dullness, and a disconnection from direction or meaning, creating the sensation of merely "going through the motions."

In women, stagnation commonly expresses as hormonal congestion, cyclical disruption, pelvic heaviness, emotional volatility, and a feeling of being energetically burdened or disconnected from intuition and creative flow. Restoring gut integrity reverses these patterns by reestablishing metabolic efficiency, hormonal balance, and neurochemical clarity, thereby rekindling vitality, sharpening perception, and restoring the embodied capacity to create, connect, and move through life with presence and purpose.

Digestive Hygiene:
Foundational Practices for Vitality

- What is digestive hygiene?
- How poor digestive habits disrupt the entire body
- Proper food combining, chewing, meal timing
- Enzyme support, hydration, and elimination rhythms
- Bathing rituals, abdominal massage, breathwork and sound healing

Digestive hygiene refers to the **consistent habits** and **ritual practices** that support the optimal function of the gut not just during a cleanse, but every day. It is how we care for our internal terrain with the same devotion we might give to skin, hair, or sacred space. When digestion is clean and efficient, the entire body operates with more ease, clarity, and energy.

Unfortunately, many people have normalized poor digestive hygiene: rushed meals, overeating, mindless snacking, emotional eating, and chronic constipation. These habits contribute to gut stagnation and lead to a slow breakdown of vitality across every system.

Why It Matters
Poor digestive hygiene can cause:

- **Slow elimination** (less than one bowel movement per day)
- **Bloating and gas**
- **Fatigue after meals**
- **Reflux or chronic burping**
- **Skin breakouts and body odor**
- **Mood swings and foggy thinking**
- **Compromised immune response**

When the digestive fire is weak, toxins accumulate. Even a clean diet can be poorly absorbed if meals are eaten in a state of stress, without proper chewing, or at the wrong times of day.

Foundations of Digestive Hygiene

These practices should become daily, rhythmic habits that signal to the body: *It is safe to receive and release.*

1. **Eat in Peace**
   Sit down. Breathe. Say a prayer or offer gratitude. Avoid phones, TV, and heavy conversation while eating.
2. **Chew Until Liquid**
   Digestion starts in the mouth. Chewing well signals enzyme release and breaks down food for better nutrient absorption.

3. **Don't Overload Your Plate**
   Eat to 80% fullness. Overeating weakens digestive fire and slows gut motility.
4. **Hydrate Wisely**
   Drink water between meals, not during. Too much liquid during meals dilutes stomach acid and enzymes.
5. **Support Elimination**
   Eliminate at least once daily. If not, use fiber, movement, warm teas, and colon support to keep the bowels open.
6. **Stay Active**
   Movement improves lymphatic flow and gut motility. Even 10–15 minutes of walking after meals can make a difference.
7. **Honor the Gut Clock**
   Eat with the body's circadian rhythm: largest meal midday, lighter meal in the evening. Avoid eating late at night.
8. **Herbal Hygiene**
   Bitters before meals, teas to soothe or stimulate digestion, and seasonal cleansing with parasite or detox blends can all support regularity.

Ritualizing the Body

Digestive hygiene is not just about function—it is a sacred offering. Bathing the gut in warmth, care, and rhythm is a way of aligning the body with nature. When we make digestion a conscious ritual, we create room for healing not only on the physical level, but also mentally, emotionally, and spiritually.

The Lymphatic & Parasite Connection

- Parasite exposure and its systemic effects
- Lymphatic stagnation and immune overload
- The role of herbal support in moving waste
- Signs you need a cleanse
- Emotional and energetic signatures of stagnation

A healthy gut does not exist in isolation! It is part of a larger system of detoxification and protection. Two often-overlooked players in this system are the lymphatic system and parasites. When the gut becomes stagnant, both of these systems are impacted, leading to deeper dysfunction that often presents in subtle or chronic ways.

The Lymphatic System: The Silent River

The lymphatic system is the body's drainage network. It clears cellular waste, toxins, and pathogens from tissues and helps regulate the immune system. Unlike the bloodstream, it has no central pump. The lymphatic system relies purely on movement, hydration, and healthy elimination to stay flowing. When digestion is sluggish, the lymph becomes congested.

Signs of lymphatic stagnation include:

- Swollen or tender lymph nodes
- Puffy face, especially around the eyes
- Chronic sinus congestion or excessive mucus production
- Skin eruptions, rashes, acne, or dull complexion
- Breast tenderness or fibrocystic tissue
- Fatigue, heaviness, or brain fog
- Frequent infections or prolonged recovery from illness
- Cold hands and feet or poor circulation
- Weight gain or resistance to weight loss, particularly in lymph-dense areas
- Headaches, pressure sensations, or generalized inflammatory discomfort

Male-specific signs of lymphatic stagnation

- **Testicular heaviness or dull ache**, often intermittent and unexplained
- **Pelvic or perineal pressure**, especially with prolonged sitting
- **Prostate congestion symptoms**, including urinary hesitancy, weak stream, or nocturia
- **Lower abdominal or groin swelling**, reflecting impaired pelvic lymph drainage
- **Reduced libido not explained by testosterone levels alone**, often paired with fatigue or brain fog
- **Slower recovery after exercise or illness**, indicating impaired lymphatic immune transport

Female-specific signs of lymphatic stagnation

- **Pelvic heaviness or fullness**, reflecting impaired lymphatic drainage within the pelvic basin and reproductive organs
- **Breast swelling or tenderness**, due to lymph congestion and reduced clearance of estrogen metabolites
- **Cyclical lymph congestion around the menstrual cycle**, as hormonal shifts increase fluid retention and inflammatory load
- **Fluid retention in hips or thighs**, common lymph-dense regions where excess fluid and metabolic waste accumulate
- **Recurrent pelvic inflammation**, associated with immune dysregulation and chronic inflammatory signaling
- **Heightened premenstrual discomfort**, resulting from compounded hormonal congestion, fluid retention, and reduced detoxification capacity

Because a large portion of the lymphatic system surrounds the intestines, known as the *gut-associated lymphoid tissue (GALT)*, digestive stagnation has a direct and profound effect on lymphatic flow and immune surveillance. When intestinal motility is impaired, lymph circulation slows, allowing inflammatory mediators, microbial byproducts, and metabolic waste to accumulate rather than be efficiently cleared. This congestion delays detoxification, increases workload placed on the liver, compromises immune regulation, and ultimately leaves the body more vulnerable to chronic infection, inflammatory conditions, and autoimmune dysregulation.

Parasites: The Unseen Disruptors

Parasites aren't just a concern in developing countries, they are far more common than many realize. Poor elimination, travel, contaminated water or food, and even emotional or spiritual stagnation can create an internal environment where parasites thrive.

Parasite exposure can come from various sources:

- **Contaminated water or food**: Drinking untreated water or eating undercooked meat (especially pork, beef, and fish) can introduce parasites into the gut.
- **Poor hygiene**: Washing hands improperly or touching contaminated surfaces, especially in public spaces like public restrooms or public transport.
- **Travel to areas with less sanitation**: Traveling to places where water quality or food hygiene standards are less stringent can expose you to parasites, especially in developing countries.

- **Pets and animals**: Animals, particularly cats and dogs, can harbor parasites and transfer them to humans through fur or contact with feces.
- **Unwashed fruits and vegetables**: Produce that hasn't been thoroughly washed or handled can carry parasitic eggs.
- **Insect bites**: Certain parasites can enter the body through bites from infected insects such as sandflies , mosquitos and ticks as an example.
- **Emotionally or spiritually stagnant environments**: Emotional distress or unresolved trauma may create an internal environment that's more conducive to parasitic activity, where the body's defenses are weakened.

Detox Isn't A Trend:
What Real Detoxification Requires

- Phases of Detoxification
- Key herbs for gut movement, parasites, and lymph
- Preparation methods: teas, tinctures, baths, poultices
- Safety and considerations

"Detox" has become a buzzword, often reduced to green juices, teas, or quick cleanses. But true detoxification is not about deprivation. It is a complex, biological process your body is always engaged in. The key is to support, not override, this natural system.

At the heart of real detox is the liver, the body's master filter. But for detox to be successful and sustainable, multiple organs and systems including the colon, kidneys, lungs, skin, and lymph must also be supported.

The Three Phases of Detoxification

Detoxification is not a single action or event. It is a sequential, metabolically demanding process that unfolds in three interconnected phases. Each phase relies on specific nutrients, enzymes, and elimination pathways to function effectively. When any phase is unsupported or overwhelmed, detoxification becomes inefficient and can exacerbate symptoms rather than relieve them.

Phase 1: Activation (Modification)

In Phase 1, the liver identifies toxins and begins the process of chemical modification. Through enzyme systems primarily driven by the cytochrome P450 pathway, fat-soluble toxins are transformed into intermediate compounds. While this step is essential, these intermediates are often more reactive and potentially damaging than the original toxins.

Substances processed during Phase 1 include:

- Environmental chemicals such as pesticides and heavy metals
- Medications and alcohol
- Excess or spent hormones
- Metabolic waste products

This phase requires significant nutritional and antioxidant support, including:

- **B vitamins** (especially B2, B3, B6, B9, and B12) to fuel enzymatic activity
- **Antioxidants** such as vitamin C, vitamin E, and glutathione to neutralize free radicals
- **Flavonoids and plant compounds** that modulate enzyme activity and reduce oxidative stress

Without adequate antioxidant protection, Phase 1 activity can lead to increased inflammation, oxidative damage, headaches, nausea, fatigue, irritability, or a general worsening of symptoms during cleansing. This is often why individuals feel unwell during poorly supported detox protocols.

Phase 2: Conjugation (Neutralization)

Phase 2 is the body's primary protective phase. Here, the reactive intermediates produced in Phase 1 are bound to specific molecules that render them less toxic and water-soluble, allowing for safe elimination.

This neutralization process depends heavily on:

- **Amino acids** such as glycine, taurine, cysteine, and methionine

- **Sulfur-containing compounds**, commonly found in garlic, onions, and cruciferous vegetables
- **Glutathione**, the body's master antioxidant and detoxifier
- **Herbs that support liver conjugation**, including burdock root, dandelion root, and milk thistle

When Phase 2 is under-resourced or sluggish, toxins processed in Phase 1 cannot be safely neutralized. Instead, they may accumulate or recirculate, contributing to symptoms such as skin eruptions, rashes, hormonal disruption, mood instability, headaches, and chemical sensitivity.

Phase 3: Elimination (Transport and Excretion)

Phase 3 is the exit phase of detoxification. Once toxins have been neutralized, they must be physically removed from the body through functioning elimination pathways.

Primary routes include:

- The colon, via bile secretion and stool
- The kidneys, via urine
- The lungs, via respiration
- The skin, via sweat

Effective elimination requires:

- Regular bowel movements

- Adequate hydration
- Sufficient dietary fiber
- Physical movement and sweating

If these pathways are compromised due to constipation, dehydration, poor bile flow, sedentary lifestyle, or impaired lymphatic circulation, detoxification stalls. In such cases, toxins may be reabsorbed into circulation, placing renewed burden on the liver and perpetuating systemic inflammation.

Clinical Integration

True detoxification is successful only when all three phases are supported simultaneously. Activating detox without adequate neutralization or elimination increases toxicity rather than resolving it. Sustainable detox protocols must therefore emphasize preparation, nutrient sufficiency, digestive motility, and ongoing elimination to restore balance rather than overwhelm the system.

Note on why aggressive cleanses often fail

One of the most common mistakes in detoxification is activating the detox pathways without adequately supporting neutralization and elimination. Aggressive cleanses that rely heavily on stimulants, fasting, or high-dose detox agents may rapidly increase Phase 1 activity while leaving Phase 2 and Phase 3 under-resourced. When this occurs, toxins are mobilized faster than the body can safely process and remove them.

This imbalance often results in a worsening of symptoms rather than improvement. Individuals may experience headaches, nausea, fatigue, skin eruptions, hormonal disruption, anxiety, or emotional volatility. These reactions are frequently misinterpreted as "detox symptoms," when in reality they reflect toxic recirculation and physiological overload rather than effective cleansing.

Sustainable detoxification requires preparation, adequate nutrition, hydration, bowel regularity, and lymphatic support. Without these foundations, detox efforts can place excessive strain on the liver, nervous system, and immune response. For this reason, successful recalibration prioritizes balance, sequencing, and replenishment over speed or intensity.

Supporting All Phases for a True Reset

A true detox program supports all three phases:

- **Preparation phase**: Begin with hydration, fiber, gentle lymphatic movement, and gut cleansing (like hydro-colonics or oral colonics).
- **Active detox phase**: Use herbs and nutrition that promote liver function, parasite cleansing, and lymphatic drainage.
- **Rebuilding phase**: Focus on restoring gut flora, nourishing the endocrine system, and stabilizing energy and mood.

When these phases are respected and supported, detox becomes a powerful process of clarity, cellular renewal, and spiritual recalibration not just weight loss or symptom suppression.

Herbal Allies for Detox & Recalibration

When the goal is recalibrating the body physically, emotionally, spiritually herbs become sacred allies. They gently nudge the systems back into rhythm, support waste elimination, and help reawaken the body's innate healing intelligence.

Working With Herbs in a Cleanse

- **Start gently** – Begin with lymphatic and digestive herbs before antiparasitics
- **Rotate herbs** – Especially for parasites, to avoid resistance and stagnation
- **Support all exits** – Colon, skin, kidneys, lungs, and emotional expression
- **Pair herbs with practices** – Movement, hydration, dry brushing, and breathwork enhance their effect

The Role of Herbal Support in Moving Waste

Herbs have been central to waste elimination in traditional healing systems across the globe. When used with intention and knowledge, they can:

- Stimulate lymphatic flow
- Increase bile production
- Support liver detoxification
- Promote bowel regularity
- Enhance elimination through urine, sweat, and stool

Here are key categories of herbs and their roles:

Lymphatic Movers

These herbs help move stagnation from the interstitial spaces and support the immune system:

- **Red root** (*Ceanothus americanus*) – decongests lymph nodes, especially helpful for pelvic and breast lymph
- **Cleavers** (*Galium aparine*) – gentle and cooling, excellent for surface lymph flow
- **Echinacea** (*Echinacea purpurea* also commonly *E. angustifolia, E. pallida*) – stimulates lymph movement and immune response
- **Calendula** (*Calendula officinalis*)– supports lymphatic drainage and skin detoxification

Bitters & Hepatics (Liver & Bile Support)

These herbs improve digestion, stimulate bile (which helps eliminate fat-soluble toxins), and support liver Phase I/II detox:

- **Dandelion root** (*Taraxacum officinale*) – liver detoxifier and mild laxative
- **Burdock root** (*Arctium lappa*) – purifies blood, supports liver and kidneys
- **Milk thistle** (*Silybum marianum*) – protects and regenerates liver cells
- **Yellow dock** (*Rumex crispus*) – bitter and iron-rich, promotes bowel regularity

Antiparasitics & Antimicrobials

These herbs directly target pathogens and support microbial balance:

- **Wormwood** (*Artemisia absinthium*) – potent antiparasitic, best used in formulas
- **Black walnut hull** (*Juglans nigra* (green hull) – cleanses parasites and fungal overgrowth
- **Clove** (*Syzygium aromaticum*) – helps kill parasite eggs and has broad antimicrobial effects
- **Garlic** (*Allium sativum*) – immune support, anti-parasitic, and gut microbiome friendly

Diuretics & Diaphoretics

- **Nettle leaf** (*Urtica dioica*) – flushes toxins via the kidneys
- **Yarrow** (*Achillea millefolium*) – induces sweating and supports circulation
- **Corn silk** (*Zea mays* (stigma) – soothes and supports urinary elimination
- **Dandelion Root** (*Taraxacum officinale)*- enhances the elimination of metabolic waste through both the digestive and urinary systems

Key Herbs by Focus

For Gut Movement & Digestion

- **Senna** (*Senna alexandrina*) – stimulant laxative; short-term use only
- **Slippery elm** (*Ulmus rubra*) – soothes inflamed gut, supports elimination
- **Marshmallow root** (*Althaea officinalis*) – moistens and coats the digestive tract
- **Ginger** (*Zingiber officinale*) – increases digestive fire, reduces gas and stagnation

For Parasite Detox

- **Wormwood** (*Artemisia absinthium*) – antiparasitic, bitter tonic
- **Black walnut hull** (*Juglans nigra*) – antifungal, anti-worm properties
- **Clove** (*Syzygium aromaticum*) – targets parasite eggs, antimicrobial
- **Neem** (*Azadirachta indica*) – blood purifier, antifungal, anti-worm

For Lymphatic & Liver Support

- **Red root** (*Ceanothus americanus*) – moves stagnant lymph
- **Cleavers** (*Galium aparine*) – cooling, lymph-moving herb
- **Milk thistle** (*Silybum marianum*) – supports liver detox and regeneration

- **Burdock root** (*Arctium lappa*) – purifies blood, supports liver, lymph, and skin
- **Yellow dock** (*Rumex crispus*) – bitter, mild laxative, iron-rich

Preparation Methods: Different herbs work best with different forms of preparation. Below are some basic methods:

Teas (Infusions & Decoctions)

- Best for leaves, flowers, soft roots
- Example: Cleavers + nettle infusion for lymph and minerals
- Simmer harder roots (burdock, yellow dock) as decoctions

Tinctures

- Alcohol or glycerin-based extracts for longer shelf life
- Ideal for potent herbs like black walnut, wormwood, or milk thistle
- Use drop doses (especially antiparasitic herbs)

Baths & Steams

- Herbal baths allow for skin detoxification and relaxation
- Use epsom salts + calendula, ginger, or rosemary
- Vaginal steams (yoni steams) may support lymphatic drainage in pelvic region

Poultices & Oils

- Topical application for swollen lymph nodes or skin detox
- Example: Castor oil packs over liver or abdomen to support elimination

Safety & Considerations

- **Start slow:** Too much too soon can overwhelm elimination pathways
- **Stay hydrated:** Herbs are helpers, but water is the carrier
- **Track reactions:** Detox can surface emotional or physical shifts
- **Use breaks:** Some herbs, especially antiparasitics, should be pulsed (e.g., 3 days on, 2 days off)
- **Contraindications:** Always consider pregnancy, medications, or pre-existing conditions

The 21-Day Reset Protocol

The **21-Day Reset** is a sacred container of rest, release, and realignment. Rooted in over a decade of practice, this protocol is not just about detoxing the body, it's about recalibrating the self on all levels: physical, emotional, energetic, and spiritual.

This reset was designed to eliminate common dietary and energetic disruptions while promoting gut cleansing, parasite elimination, system rebalance/reset and the reawakening of vitality and clarity. It invites participants to slow down, listen inward, and reconnect with their original blueprint of wellness.

Reset Commitments

Foods to Avoid:

- No meat (nothing that had parents)
- No dairy (includes eggs)
- No sweets or processed sugars
- No breads or pasta
- No white potatoes

- No white rice
- No alcohol, coffee, sodas
- No smoking (cigarettes , cigars , vaping , hookah, etc.) (ritual use excluded)
- No recreational drug use

Energetic & Behavioral Guidelines:

- No sex (physical or oral) , kissing, or unnecessary touching
- No cursing or gossip
- No excessive social media use (If you can do no social media that would be optimal
- No music , tv programs that have low vibrational, destructive, abusive or spiritually/emotionally jaunting themes
- Wear all white, both under and outer garments, to promote clarity and spiritual neutrality (If work uniform is not white , where white underneath uniform)
- Change bed sheets to solid colors, preferably white or pale colors. No patterns, black or red sheets. This also applies to towels for bathing

What to Increase:

- Fruits, vegetables, legumes and whole grains
- Clean water and fresh juices
- Physical movement and exercise
- Sunlight and fresh air
- Yoni / Lingham Steams

Daily Practices

- **Morning Prayer** at sunrise (or as close to sunrise as possible) to set intention and align with spirit
- **Evening Meditation** to the ancestors give thanks, ask for guidance, and reflect on the day
- **Daily Bathing Ritual** using African black soap and a loofah sponge to cleanse the physical and energetic body
- **Journaling** every day to track physical changes, emotional releases, and spiritual insights

Colon Support & Cleansing Schedule

A clean gut is foundational to this reset. The following schedule supports deep intestinal cleansing:

- **Day 1:** Hydro-colon therapy (or oral colonic if unavailable)
- **Day 15:** Hydro-colon therapy (or oral colonic if unavailable)
- **Day 22:** Hydro-colon therapy (optional but recommended)

These sessions clear impacted/calcified waste, mucus, and parasite nests that impair digestion and absorption. Many participants report improved clarity, sleep, and bowel function afterward.

The third hydrocolon therapy session on Day 22 is considered optional because, by this point in the reset, many individuals have already achieved improved bowel motility and effective elimination through dietary changes, hydration, herbal support, and the first two sessions. For those who are experiencing regular, complete bowel movements and a sense of digestive relief, additional mechanical cleansing may not be necessary. However, the optional session can provide added support for individuals who continue to experience sluggish elimination, residual bloating, or a sense of incomplete clearing as they transition out of the reset and into the nourishment phase.

Why These Practices Are Avoided During the Reset

1. **No sex (physical or oral), kissing, or unnecessary touching:** Sexual and intimate contact involves significant energetic, hormonal, and physiological exchange. During a reset, abstaining from sexual activity conserves vital energy, reduces neuroendocrine stimulation, and limits fluid exchange at a time when the body is actively mobilizing and eliminating toxins, metabolic waste, hormones, and inflammatory byproducts. Sexual activity redirects blood flow, lymphatic movement, and nervous system signaling away from detoxification and tissue repair, potentially interrupting the clearing process and increasing the redistribution of mobilized waste.

Root & Recalibrate

Abstinence allows the body to prioritize internal cleansing, stabilize hormonal signaling, and complete detoxification without interruption. In men, this period of sexual restraint supports reproductive health by conserving zinc, amino acids, and other nutrients essential for sperm production, improving seminal quality, and reducing oxidative stress that can impair fertility. When practiced consciously as a couple, temporary sexual abstinence can also deepen relational intimacy by shifting connection away from physical release and toward presence, breath, emotional attunement, and shared intention. This creates space for a more tantric form of intimacy rooted in energetic coherence, mutual regulation, and intentional bonding rather than performance or physical fulfillment alone.

It is important to note that this practice is not about suppression, rejection, or deprivation, but about timing and intentional redirection of energy in service of healing. Couples are encouraged to replace sexual activity with shared grounding practices such as synchronized breathing, holding hands in stillness, eye contact, prayer or meditation together, gentle walking, or preparing meals side by side with intention. These practices support nervous system regulation, preserve connection, and often lead to a deeper sense of closeness that enhances intimacy once physical union is reintroduced after the reset.

2. **No cursing or gossip**: Speech carries both psychological and physiological impact. Negative or reactive language activates stress pathways, elevates cortisol, and reinforces mental agitation. Avoiding cursing and gossip supports nervous system regulation, emotional clarity, and intentional communication during a period of heightened sensitivity and internal focus.

3. **No excessive social media use (ideally none)** Excessive social media exposure overstimulates the nervous system, disrupts circadian rhythm, and fragments attention through constant comparison, emotional reactivity, and dopamine-driven engagement. Reducing or eliminating social media supports mental quiet, emotional grounding and deeper awareness of bodily cues during detoxification.

4. **No music or television with low-vibrational, destructive, abusive, or emotionally jarring themes**: Sensory input directly influences the nervous system and emotional state. Exposure to violent, chaotic, or emotionally dysregulating content can activate stress responses and counteract the calming, restorative processes required for healing. Choosing neutral or uplifting sensory input supports nervous system stability, emotional safety, and spiritual clarity throughout the reset.

Why the White Clothing?

Wearing white from head to toe acts as both a visual and energetic commitment to purification. In color therapy, white is understood as the integration of all colors, symbolizing wholeness, neutrality, and reset. Because white reflects light rather than absorbing it, it is associated with mental clarity, heightened awareness, and energetic containment.

On a psychological level, wearing white reduces visual noise and external stimulation, helping to quiet the nervous system and support introspection. Energetically, white is traditionally used across spiritual systems as a protective and consecrating color, reinforcing boundaries and accountability in thought, speech, and behavior. Within the context of this reset, white clothing serves as a constant somatic reminder to move with clarity, restraint, and sacred intention as the body and spirit recalibrate.

Yoni and Lingam Steams: Parasite, Lymphatic, and Hormonal Support

During the reset, yoni and lingam steams may be used as targeted, non-invasive practices to support pelvic detoxification without external fluid exchange. Gentle steam increases localized circulation and lymphatic movement in the pelvic basin, an area rich in lymph nodes and hormone-responsive tissues. This enhanced flow supports the mobilization and drainage of stagnant fluids, inflammatory byproducts, and microbial debris, creating an environment less favorable for parasitic persistence while improving immune surveillance.

Steaming also supports hormonal regulation by improving tissue perfusion and assisting the clearance of spent hormones and inflammatory metabolites from uterine, vaginal, prostatic, and perineal tissues. When paired with overall gut and liver support, these practices can help reduce pelvic congestion, ease cyclical discomfort, and promote balanced endocrine signaling during detoxification.

Timing Guidelines During the Reset:

- **Frequency:** 1–2 steams (or more if steaming for pathology) times per week during the 21-day reset
- **Best timing:** In the evening, after the day's main elimination activities (bowel movement, hydration, gentle movement)
- **Duration:** 15–25 minutes per session
- **For women:** Avoid steaming during active menstruation; resume post-menses if desired

- **For men:** Steams may be used consistently throughout the reset, focusing on gentle warmth rather than intensity

Steaming should feel soothing and restorative, not stimulating or depleting. When used intentionally and in moderation, yoni and lingam steams complement parasite balance, lymphatic drainage, and hormonal recalibration while preserving energetic boundaries and allowing the body to remain oriented toward internal cleansing and repair.

When used alongside gut and liver support, yoni and lingam steams act as adjunct Phase 3 elimination practices by enhancing pelvic circulation and lymphatic drainage, thereby supporting the localized clearance of inflammatory byproducts, spent hormones, and microbial debris during detoxification.

Integration of Herbal Support

Throughout the reset, you may incorporate supportive herbal teas that assist:

- **Lymphatic drainage**
- **Parasite elimination**
- **Liver and gallbladder detoxification**

- **Nervous system support** (especially during days of emotional clearing)

These blends are not mandatory, but deeply enhance the results when used consistently with clean water and whole foods.

This protocol is not a punishment or restriction. It is a return to center, a recalibration of your entire being. Many who have completed the 21-Day Reset report:

- Better digestion and elimination
- Deeper sleep and more vivid dreams
- Renewed sexual vitality and spiritual sensitivity
- Clarity of thought, intention, and life direction

Up next, we'll explore how to maintain and build on the gains of the reset, and how it aligns with the body's seasonal and energetic rhythms.

Spiritual & Energetic Detoxification

- The impact of emotional residue and spiritual stagnation
- Ancestor connection, prayer, breath, ritual bathing
- Importance of sexual discipline and energetic boundaries
- Plant spirit allies and spiritual hygiene tools

True healing is not complete without addressing the spiritual and energetic bodies. Just as the gut can become congested with waste, our spirit can hold on to grief, trauma, emotional residue, and energetic debris. These unseen blockages often weigh down vitality, cloud intuition, and prevent alignment with our highest self.

This part of the detox journey honors the unseen.

The Impact of Emotional Residue & Spiritual Stagnation

Unprocessed emotions such as anger, fear, grief, guilt, and resentment do not simply disappear when ignored or suppressed. Instead, they often become physiologically embedded, influencing nervous system tone, hormonal signaling, immune responsiveness, and digestive function. When emotions are not expressed, witnessed, or integrated, they can persist as emotional residue, subtly shaping bodily patterns and energetic flow over time.

From a neurobiological perspective, unresolved emotional experiences are encoded within the limbic system, particularly the amygdala and hippocampus, which govern emotional memory and threat perception. When these experiences remain unprocessed, the nervous system may stay in a heightened or dysregulated state, characterized by elevated cortisol levels and reduced parasympathetic (vagal) tone. This chronic activation disrupts gut–brain communication, alters digestive secretions and motility, impairs sleep architecture, and weakens immune regulation.

Over time, this emotional residue may:

- **Weaken immune function** by sustaining low-grade stress responses that impair immune surveillance and tissue repair
- **Disrupt digestion and sleep** through persistent sympathetic nervous system activation and altered circadian signaling

- **Manifest as chronic fatigue, anxiety, or low mood**, reflecting prolonged neuroendocrine and neurotransmitter imbalance
- **Create energetic congestion**, experienced as mental fog, loss of direction, emotional heaviness, or spiritual disconnection

From both a clinical and spiritual perspective, emotional stagnation mirrors physical stagnation. Just as retained waste burdens the body's detoxification systems, unresolved emotional material occupies psychological and energetic space, limiting clarity, intuition, and vitality.

During detoxification, as inflammatory burden decreases and parasympathetic tone improves, the nervous system gains the capacity to safely process previously suppressed emotional content. Memories, sensations, or emotional waves may surface unexpectedly. This emergence is not a sign of regression or instability; rather, it reflects the body's innate intelligence recognizing sufficient safety and support for release. When met with presence, compassion, and intentional practice, emotional release becomes an essential component of healing and holistic recalibration.

Ancestor Connection, Prayer, and Breath

Detoxification becomes sacred when it is approached not only as a physical process, but as a relational one a dialogue between body, spirit, and lineage. When practiced in communion with spirit, cleansing transforms from an act of removal into an act of remembrance, alignment, and restoration.

- **Prayer at sunrise** anchors the day in intention and gratitude, aligning the body's rhythms with natural cycles of light and renewal. Morning prayer helps regulate cortisol, centers the mind, and establishes a conscious orientation toward healing before the demands of the day take hold. It creates a spiritual container in which detoxification can unfold with purpose rather than strain.
- **Breathwork** serves as a bridge between the conscious and unconscious body. Slow, intentional breathing increases oxygen delivery to tissues, stimulates lymphatic movement, and activates the parasympathetic nervous system, signaling safety and rest. Through breath, stagnant emotional and energetic patterns begin to loosen, allowing both physical toxins and emotional residue to move without force.
- **Ancestral reverence**, practiced through candle lighting, offerings, prayer, or altar time,

reconnects the individual to an unbroken lineage of survival, wisdom, and resilience. During periods of detox and vulnerability, this connection provides grounding and protection, reminding the practitioner that release is supported by those who came before. Honoring ancestors during cleansing reinforces continuity and strength as old patterns, burdens, and inherited imprints are consciously released.

- **Sound therapy**, including drumming, chanting, humming, singing bowls, or ancestral music, supports neuroregulation by gently synchronizing brainwave activity and calming the nervous system. Sound bypasses cognitive processing and works directly on the limbic system, helping ease emotional tension, reduce stress responses, and create a sense of internal coherence during detoxification.

Even five minutes of intentional stillness at the beginning and end of each day can recalibrate the inner compass. These moments of quiet presence allow the nervous system to settle, the spirit to orient, and the body to integrate the work of cleansing with clarity, safety, and reverence.

Zaire Sabb, PhD(C)

Sexual Discipline, Sacral Regulation, and Vagal Tone

Sexual energy is a concentrated expression of life force that interfaces directly with the sacral center, the autonomic nervous system, and endocrine signaling. During detoxification, abstaining from sexual contact, including kissing and excessive touch, supports the downregulation of sympathetic arousal and the restoration of parasympathetic dominance, a state necessary for digestion, detoxification, immune repair, and emotional integration.

From a neurobiological perspective, sexual stimulation activates dopaminergic and oxytocin-mediated reward pathways while simultaneously engaging the vagus nerve, which governs gut motility, inflammatory regulation, heart rate variability, and emotional regulation. While these pathways are beneficial in appropriate contexts, frequent stimulation during detox can fragment nervous system signaling and divert physiological resources away from restoration. Sexual discipline allows vagal tone to stabilize, supporting coherent gut–brain communication and improving the body's capacity to process both physical toxins and emotional residue.

Sacral Center Integrity and Energetic Containment

The sacral center governs creativity, reproduction, emotional fluidity, and relational exchange. During periods of chronic stress, illness, or energetic depletion, this center may become dysregulated, resulting in scattered focus, emotional volatility, diminished libido, or compulsive seeking of external stimulation. Temporarily withdrawing from sexual and intimate exchange allows the sacral center to rebuild integrity, restoring internal rhythm, containment, and creative vitality.

This practice matters because it:

- **Consolidates life force**, enhancing clarity, presence, and embodied awareness
- **Supports sacral recalibration**, improving emotional regulation and creative flow
- **Protects energetic boundaries**, preventing unnecessary depletion or entanglement during heightened sensitivity

Semen Retention and Physiological Replenishment

In men, temporary semen retention during detox supports metabolic and neurological conservation rather than loss. Semen contains high concentrations of zinc, amino acids, fatty acids, and signaling compounds essential for immune function, testosterone synthesis, and nervous system stability. Frequent ejaculation during periods of detox may increase nutrient demand and neuroendocrine fluctuation at a time when the body is prioritizing elimination and repair.

Short-term retention supports:

- **Nutrient conservation**, particularly zinc and B vitamins
- **Hormonal stabilization**, reducing excessive prolactin and post-ejaculatory fatigue
- **Improved autonomic balance**, supporting parasympathetic dominance and vagal regulation
- **Enhanced vitality and focus**, as metabolic resources are redirected toward healing rather than reproductive output

Importantly, this practice is not framed as suppression, denial, or moral restriction, but as intentional containment in service of restoration.

Energetic Boundaries and Nervous System Safety

Energetic boundaries extend beyond sexual contact. Emotional dumping, over-giving, and absorbing others' stressors activate threat-based nervous system responses that undermine detoxification. During recalibration, maintaining clear interpersonal boundaries preserves nervous system safety, reduces cortisol load, and supports emotional coherence.

Wearing white throughout the reset reinforces these boundaries both symbolically and somatically. As a reflective, neutral color, white supports containment and clarity while acting as a continual reminder to move with restraint, intention, and reverence as the nervous system, sacral center, and energetic field stabilize.

Female Parallel: Ovulatory and Luteal Phase Sensitivity

In women, sexual discipline during detox also supports nervous system regulation and hormonal stability, particularly during the ovulatory and luteal phases of the menstrual cycle, when the body is more sensitive to stimulation, fluid shifts, and emotional input. Ovulation represents a peak in estrogen and energetic outward expression, while the luteal phase is characterized by increased progesterone demand, heightened nervous system sensitivity, and a greater need for rest, containment, and internal resource conservation.

During these phases, sexual activity and intense

relational exchange can amplify fluid movement, lymphatic load, and neuroendocrine fluctuations at a time when the body is already managing hormonal transitions and detoxification processes. Temporarily abstaining allows metabolic and nervous system resources to remain directed toward liver detoxification, progesterone support, and parasympathetic regulation rather than outward expenditure.

From a sacral and vagal perspective, sexual discipline during ovulation and the luteal phase supports:

- **Stabilization of vagal tone**, improving digestion, emotional regulation, and sleep quality
- **Reduction of pelvic and lymphatic congestion**, particularly in the uterus, ovaries, and breast tissue
- **Improved hormonal clearance**, assisting the elimination of spent estrogens and inflammatory metabolites
- **Emotional containment**, reducing premenstrual irritability, anxiety, or emotional overwhelm

This practice is not about suppression of desire, but about honoring cyclical physiology and allowing the reproductive and nervous systems to recalibrate without excessive stimulation. By conserving energy during hormonally sensitive phases, women often experience improved cycle regularity, reduced premenstrual symptoms, and a deeper sense of embodied clarity and intuition.

Clinical Note: When Sexual Abstinence May Not Be Appropriate

While temporary sexual abstinence can be supportive during detoxification and recalibration, it is not universally indicated for all individuals or circumstances. In some cases, prolonged abstinence may increase stress, emotional dysregulation, or relational strain, particularly for individuals with a history of trauma, attachment disruption, or anxiety where safe intimacy supports nervous system regulation rather than depletes it.

Sexual connection may also be appropriate when it is mutual, emotionally regulated, non-draining, and does not involve excessive stimulation or fluid exchange, especially for individuals who experience improved mood, sleep, or vagal tone through healthy relational bonding. Additionally, abstinence may be contraindicated in cases where it exacerbates obsessive thought patterns, shame responses, or physiological tension.

As with all aspects of this reset, sexual discipline should be intentional rather than rigid, responsive to individual physiology, emotional needs, and relational context. The guiding principle is whether intimacy supports restoration and regulation or contributes to depletion and dysregulation. When approached with awareness, flexibility, and consent, adjustments may be made to honor both healing and holistic well-being.

Plant Spirit Allies & Spiritual Hygiene Tools

Plants are not just physical medicine they are sentient beings with spiritual intelligence.

Spiritual allies may include:

- **White sage** (*Salvia apiana*) – clarity, purification (ethically sourced or grown)
- **Frankincense resin** – uplifts spirit, clears low vibrations
- **Rue** (*Ruta graveolens*) – breaks hexes and dense emotional attachments
- **Blue vervain** (*Verbena hastata*) – for spiritual grief and emotional repression
- **Florida Water** or traditional herbal waters – for energetic cleansing and ritual baths

Practices to integrate:

- **Herbal spiritual baths** (e.g., basil, hyssop, rosemary) for clearing and blessing
- **Smudging or fumigation** of your body and space

- **Sound healing** (drumming, singing bowls, ancestral music)
- **Journaling** after meditation to track emotional or spiritual breakthroughs

Spiritual detox isn't about perfection it's about presence. As you clean the body, give your spirit a seat at the table. The more you create stillness and intention, the more space you create for divine clarity, healing, and rebirth.

Integration After the Reset

- Transitioning out of the reset
- Integrating new habits into daily life
- Recipes, lifestyle tips, and long-term herbal support
- Journaling prompts and intention-setting

The 21-day reset is a profound journey, a time to shed the old and make space for the new. But the true magic lies not just in the detoxification process, but in how you integrate what you've learned and experienced. The transition back to daily life, after having given your body, mind, and spirit a deep reset, requires care and intention.

This section offers guidance on how to gracefully reintroduce foods, habits, and environments, while continuing to nurture the reset work you've begun.

How to Transition After the 21 Days

Coming out of the reset phase can feel like a breath of fresh air, but it can also feel overwhelming. The key is to ease back into your routine while staying mindful of your body's needs.

Root & Recalibrate

1. Slow and Steady Reintroduction

When you've completed the reset, it's important to slowly reintroduce foods and activities that were previously avoided. Start with one new food or habit at a time. Observe how your body reacts, and stay present with your emotions, energy levels, and digestion.

2. Gradual Reintroduction of Foods

- Begin by adding light, whole foods that nourish the gut, such as steamed vegetables, cooked grains, and mild proteins like fish or chicken.
- Reintroduce dairy, gluten, and processed foods only after a week or two, allowing time for your digestive system to maintain balance.
- Monitor any signs of bloating, fatigue, or inflammation, and adjust accordingly.

3. Gentle Reintroduction of Habits

- If you're returning to work or family life, practice mindful breathing **or** grounding techniques (such as placing your feet on the earth) to keep your energy in check.
- **Exercise** should be gentle focus on yoga, walking, or swimming rather than intense cardio or heavy lifting, which can put strain on the lymphatic system.

Continuing Gut, Lymph, and Emotional Care

The reset doesn't have to end after 21 days. This is a lifestyle one that requires ongoing care and nourishment.

1. Gut Health Support

- **Fiber-rich foods** (vegetables, fruits, legumes, nuts, seeds) are essential to continue nourishing the gut microbiome and promoting digestion.
- Incorporate **fermented foods** (like sauerkraut, kimchi, kombucha) to support gut flora and improve nutrient absorption.
- Consider **digestive bitters** before meals to stimulate gastric juices and enhance digestion.

2. Lymphatic System Maintenance

- Drink plenty of **water** (ideally with a pinch of sea salt for electrolytes) to keep the lymph fluid moving.
- Continue to support your lymphatic system with **light movement** like stretching, yoga, or walking.
- Massage or dry brushing the skin can stimulate lymphatic flow and prevent stagnation.

3. Emotional and Energetic Hygiene

The emotional and spiritual work you've done during the reset is an ongoing process. Make it a habit to:

- **Journal daily** about your emotional landscape and any shifts that arise.
- Stay connected to **ancestral wisdom** through prayer, ritual, or meditation.
- Continue **sexual discipline** and **energetic boundaries** to preserve your vitality.

Avoiding Rebound Toxicity

It's common to experience a "rebound" effect if old habits creep back in too quickly. The body is still in a sensitive state, and when unhealthy foods or stressors are reintroduced too soon, they can overwhelm the systems.

To avoid **rebound toxicity**:

- **Set boundaries** for yourself: create specific guidelines for reintroducing foods, and commit to them for a certain period.
- **Avoid quick fixes**: Resist the temptation to return to old habits (fast food, sugar, alcohol, etc.) in response to stress or cravings.
- **Stay grounded in your practices**: Continue meditation, journaling, and breathwork as emotional support systems, even after the reset period ends.

Moving Forward with Intention

The reset process is designed to be a springboard for long-term health and balance. As you reintegrate the rhythms of your daily life, carry the lessons of the 21-day reset forward with you. Stay committed to ongoing gut health, lymphatic movement, emotional care, and spiritual alignment. You're not just resetting your body you're recalibrating your life.

Conclusion:

Embracing the Cycle of Recalibration

- Honoring the cyclical nature of healing
- Encouragement for continued self-realignment
- Final prayer or affirmation

As you reach the end of this 21-day reset, it's important to honor the cyclical nature of healing. Just as the seasons ebb and flow, your body, mind, and spirit are constantly evolving. This reset is not a one-time event but the beginning of a deeper, ongoing process of self-care, renewal, and alignment.

The work you've done over the past weeks whether physical, emotional, or spiritual has helped to clear away stagnation, release toxins, and restore balance. However, healing is not linear. It's a continuous cycle of growth, shedding, and transformation. Be gentle with yourself as you continue this journey, and remember that each phase is vital for your overall well-being.

Encouragement for Continued Self-Realignment

As you move forward, stay committed to your path of self-realignment. Healing is a lifelong journey, and there will always be moments when you need to pause, reflect, and recalibrate. Trust your intuition and continue to nourish your body with whole, nourishing foods, engage in practices that support your mind and spirit, and cultivate sacred spaces for yourself in all aspects of your life.

Make time for regular cleansing whether that's through detoxification practices, journaling, or connecting with nature. Keep your energetic boundaries strong and honor your body's rhythms. The more you honor yourself, the more in tune you will be with your true essence.

Final Prayer/Affirmation

I am grounded in the truth of my being. My body is a sacred vessel, and I honor its wisdom.

I release what no longer serves me and welcome the healing that flows through me.

I trust the process of recalibration and know that every step I take brings me closer to my highest self.

I am grateful for the journey and the transformation that is unfolding in my life. With each day, I grow stronger, clearer, and more aligned with my purpose.

With love,

Z

Preparing for the 21-Day Reset & Transitioning Off the Reset

Before the 21-Day Reset: Journal Prompts

These prompts are designed to help you reflect on your current state, set intentions, and prepare mentally, physically, and spiritually for the reset.

1. **Current Health Status**
   - How do you feel in your body right now? What areas feel stagnant or unbalanced?
   - What are your primary health concerns or goals going into this reset?

2. **Emotional State**
   - What emotions have been most present in your life recently?
   - How do you feel emotionally about starting this detox? What do you hope to release?

3. **Spiritual Readiness**
   - How aligned do you feel with your spiritual practices?
   - What spiritual goals would you like to achieve during this reset?

4. **Setting Intentions**
    - What are your specific goals for the 21-day reset (physical, emotional, spiritual)?
    - What do you hope to manifest or transform by the end of the reset?

5. **Current Habits & Challenges**
    - What habits or patterns do you feel may be the most difficult to release during this reset?
    - How can you prepare yourself mentally and emotionally to tackle these challenges?

Journal Prompts for Spiritual & Energetic Detoxification

1. **Emotional Residue**
    - What emotions or past experiences have you noticed resurfacing during this detox?
    - How do these emotions relate to any patterns in your life that you're ready to release?

2. **Ancestor Connection**
    - Have you felt any connections or guidance from your ancestors throughout this process?
    - In what ways can you honor their wisdom and guidance moving forward?

3. **Spiritual Stagnation**
   - What areas of your life or energy feel stagnant or blocked right now?
   - How can you begin to address these blockages whether through prayer, ritual, or other spiritual practices?

4. **Sexual Discipline and Boundaries**
   - How has practicing sexual discipline (abstinence or conscious intimacy) impacted your energy levels and spiritual clarity?
   - What insights have you gained about your relationship with physical intimacy and energetic exchange?

5. **Energetic Boundaries**
   - Are there people or situations in your life that drain your energy?
   - How can you strengthen your boundaries to protect your vitality and maintain your spiritual health?

6. **Spiritual Hygiene Rituals**
   - What spiritual practices (ritual baths, smudging, prayer, etc.) have felt most supportive during this detox?
   - How can you incorporate these practices into your regular routine for continued energetic cleansing and protection?

7. Inner Reflection and Growth

- After completing this section of the detox, what do you feel you've released or transformed within yourself?
- What new practices, beliefs, or habits are you ready to cultivate to maintain your spiritual and energetic health?

11-Day Journal Prompts for the Reset

These prompts will guide your reflections each day during the reset, keeping you aligned with your intentions and helping you stay mindful throughout the process.

Day 1
- How do you feel about starting this reset? What are your immediate thoughts and emotions as you begin?
- What are your intentions for this detox journey?

Day 2
- Are you noticing any physical sensations or changes in your body today?
- How are you adjusting to the changes in your daily routine?

Day 3
- What emotions have come up so far during the reset?
- How are you processing and releasing them?

Day 4
- Have you noticed any shifts in your energy levels or mental clarity?

- What positive changes are you beginning to
  feel?

Day 5
- Reflect on any challenges or cravings you've
  faced. How have you managed them so far?
- What has been the hardest part of the reset?

Day 6
- How does your body feel today? What physical
  symptoms or changes have you observed?
- Are there any deeper emotional or spiritual
  shifts happening for you?

Day 7
- Reflect on the progress you've made so far.
  What are you most proud of?
- How can you celebrate these small victories
  and keep momentum going?

Day 8
- Have you felt more connected to your spiritual
  practices?
- What has been the most grounding part of your
  reset journey?

Day 9
- How are you feeling emotionally today?
- What thoughts or feelings have come up that
  may need deeper healing or attention?

Day 10

- What lessons have you learned so far?
- How have you grown mentally, physically, or spiritually over the past 10 days?

Day 11

- As the reset comes to a close, what reflections and insights have you gained about your body, mind, and spirit?
- What will you carry forward from this reset into your everyday life?

Transitioning Off the Reset:
Checklist & Journal Prompt

As you begin to transition off the 21-day reset, it's important to ease back into your routine with intention. Here's a checklist to help you do just that:

Transitioning Off the Reset: Checklist

1. **Gradually Reintroduce Foods**
   - Start with light, nourishing foods like fruits, vegetables, and grains.
   - Reintroduce meat, dairy, and processed foods slowly, paying attention to how your body reacts.
2. **Maintain Hydration**: Continue to drink plenty of water and herbal teas to support digestion and detoxification.
3. **Nourish Your Body with Gentle Movement**: Engage in light exercise, yoga, or walking to keep energy flowing and aid digestion.
4. **Continue Mindful Practices**: Keep up with journaling, meditation, and prayer as a way to stay grounded and connected.
5. **Honor Emotional and Spiritual Shifts**: Take note of any emotional changes or new spiritual insights. Allow time for reflection and integration.

- **Reflection on the Reset**

  - Looking back on the 21-day reset, what transformation have you experienced, both physically and emotionally?
  - What aspects of the reset were the most challenging, and how did you overcome them?
  - What lessons or insights will you carry forward into your daily life to maintain your health and alignment?

Spiritual Bath Recipe & Ritual

Purpose:
To cleanse emotional and energetic residue, reconnect with your higher self and ancestors, and reset your spiritual field. Best done during the first 3 days of the reset, a full moon, or after any intense emotional release.

Ingredients:

- 1 handful of dried basil (cleansing, clarity)
- 1 handful of dried rosemary (protection, remembrance)
- 1 handful of dried lemongrass (purification, grounding)
- A pinch of sea salt (energetic clearing)
- A few drops of Florida water or rosewater (optional, for softening energy)
- White candle
- A clear bowl for collecting bathwater (for disposal ritual)
- White clothing or wrap to wear after

Instructions:

1. **Prepare the herbs:**
   Boil 2–3 cups of water, add herbs, and let steep covered for 20–30 minutes. Strain and pour into your bathwater.
2. **Set the space:**
   Light your white candle. Dim the lights. You may

wish to burn incense (frankincense, myrrh, copal) or play soft ancestral music or drumming.

3. **Spoken intention (say aloud or whisper):**

   "As I enter this water, I release all that no longer serves me spiritually, emotionally, and physically. I return to myself. I invite clarity, protection, and alignment."

4. **Bathe in silence or prayer:**

   Submerge your body or pour the water over you slowly. Focus on areas of tension or stagnation. Visualize light entering and darkness being released.

5. **Close the ritual:**

   Once finished, collect a portion of the bathwater and dispose of it outside at the base of a tree or crossroads, speaking a word of gratitude.

6. **Aftercare:**

   Dress in white. Rest. Journal your insights or dreams that follow.

Breathwork Ritual for Recalibration

Purpose:
To move stagnant emotional energy, reconnect to the body, and align with spirit. This practice supports the nervous system and gut-brain connection.

Technique: *Three-Part Conscious Breath (Belly–Rib–Chest)*

Time: 5–10 minutes daily, ideally upon waking or before meditation.

Instructions:

1. **Find your seat or lie down.**
   Close your eyes. Place one hand on your belly, the other on your heart.
2. **Begin with awareness.**
   Breathe naturally for a few moments. Feel where your breath is shallow or held.
3. **Start the Three-Part Breath:**

   - **Inhale through the nose** into the belly (feel it rise),
     then into the ribs (expand outward),
     then into the chest (lift slightly).
   - **Exhale through the mouth**—release everything in reverse: chest, ribs, belly.

4. **Repeat for 7–10 cycles.**
   Keep the breath smooth and connected. Feel into

areas of tightness and let the exhale be a soft surrender.

5. Spoken intention on final breath:
> "With each breath, I return to wholeness. With each exhale, I release what I no longer need."

Optional Integration:
Lay in stillness after your breath practice and place a glass of water near your navel. This can symbolically draw out emotional density. Discard it outside afterward with intention.

Bridging

From Clearing to Cultivation

Detoxification is an act of release. Nourishment is an act of remembrance.

Throughout this reset, you have cleared stagnation from the gut, supported the lymphatic system, addressed parasitic burden, regulated the nervous system, and confronted emotional and energetic residue held within the body. You have practiced restraint, intention, and stillness. In doing so, you have created space—physically, emotionally, and spiritually.

But space alone is not the goal.

Once the body releases what no longer serves, it enters a receptive state. The tissues are more sensitive. The nervous system is more attuned. The digestive system is quieter, more discerning. In this openness, the body does not ask for more cleansing it asks to be fed wisely.

True recalibration does not end with elimination. It completes itself through replenishment. This is the moment where many healing journeys falter. Without intentional nourishment, the cleared body can drift back into depletion, instability, or overcorrection. Sustainable balance requires a shift from removal to restoration, from discipline to devotion, from detoxification to daily rhythm.

Food, when approached with presence, becomes medicine. Preparation becomes prayer. Eating becomes an act of alignment. The same awareness cultivated during this reset is now meant to live on... not as restriction, but as ritual.

The work continues, not through another cleanse, but through how you feed your blood, calm your nervous system, rebuild mineral stores, and reestablish trust between your body and spirit.

This next phase is not about rules. It is about relationship. In the pages that follow this reset, the practices of nourishment, timing, and sacred preparation take center stage. The body learns not only how to release, but how to remain whole. The path forward is one of cultivation.

Appendix

Common Signs of Parasitic Overload

Digestive & Elimination
- **Chronic bloating or abdominal distension** *(protozoa, helminths – early)*
- **Irregular bowel movements (constipation, diarrhea, or alternating patterns)** *(protozoa, helminths – early to late)*
- **Excessive gas or foul-smelling stools** *(protozoa – early)*
- **Persistent sugar or carbohydrate cravings** *(protozoa, yeast-associated parasites – early)*
- **Feeling hungry shortly after eating** *(protozoa – early)*
- **Unexplained weight loss or difficulty gaining muscle** *(helminths – late)*

Neurological, Mood & Cognitive
- **Brain fog or difficulty concentrating** *(protozoa – early)*
- **Unexplained anxiety or panic-like sensations** *(protozoa – early)*
- **Sudden mood swings or irritability** *(protozoa – early to mid)*
- **Depressive symptoms or emotional flattening** *(chronic parasitic burden – late)*
- **Tinnitus or ringing in the ears** *(protozoa, flukes – mid to late)*
- **Restless legs or internal agitation, especially at night** *(helminths – mid)*

Sleep & Circadian Clues
- **Disturbed sleep or waking between 2–4 a.m.** *(helminths, liver flukes – mid)*
- **Nightmares or unusually vivid dreams** *(helminths – mid)*
- **Bruxism (teeth grinding), especially during sleep** *(helminths – early)*
- **Insomnia with nighttime restlessness** *(protozoa, helminths – mid)*

Dermatological & Sensory
- **Anal itching or rectal discomfort, particularly at night** *(pinworms/helminths – early)*
- **Skin rashes, hives, or unexplained itching** *(protozoa, helminths – early to mid)*
- **Crawling or itching sensations on the skin without rash** *(helminths – mid)*
- **Dark circles under the eyes** *(chronic parasitic load – mid to late)*
- **Hair thinning or brittle nails** *(nutrient-depleting helminths – late)*

Immune & Systemic
- **Frequent infections or weakened immune response** *(chronic parasitic burden – mid to late)*
- **Low-grade fevers or chills without clear infection** *(protozoa – mid)*
- **Swollen lymph nodes without acute illness** *(chronic parasitic + lymphatic involvement – late)*
- **Persistent eosinophilia on bloodwork** *(helminths – mid to late)*
- **Delayed recovery from illness or exercise** *(chronic parasitic burden – late)*

Metabolic & Nutrient Clues
- **Nutrient deficiencies despite adequate intake** *(helminths – mid to late)*
- **Iron deficiency or anemia without clear cause** *(helminths – late)*
- **Cold intolerance or fatigue after meals** *(protozoa, metabolic interference – mid)*

Energetic & Functional Observations *(Commonly reported clinically; not diagnostic)*
- **Feeling "drained" or heavy after meals** *(chronic parasitic load – mid)*
- **Sudden aversion to bitter foods or cleansing herbs** *(parasite survival response – early)*
- **Symptom flares around the full moon** *(helminths – mid to late; observational)*

Clinical Note

Many intestinal parasites, most notably *Enterobius vermicularis* (pinworms), are nocturnally active, migrating to the perianal area at night to lay eggs, a process that commonly triggers itching, restlessness, and sleep disruption and serves as an important clinical clue. More broadly, parasitic overload rarely presents as a single isolated symptom and instead manifests as clusters spanning digestion, mood, immune function, sleep patterns, and nutrient status.

Early presentations are often subtle and primarily neurological or digestive in nature, while more advanced stages reflect increasing systemic burden, immune dysregulation, and progressive nutrient depletion.

Ultimately, parasites weaken gut integrity, steal nutrients, and produce toxic waste that burdens the liver and lymphatic system. They can also create biofilms, which are protective layers that shield them from the immune system and herbal interventions, making them more difficult to eliminate without focused, strategic protocols. Due to the biofilm that is created single-herb or short cleanses have a high potential to fail.

Interconnected Systems
Gut stagnation creates a physiological environment in which parasites are more likely to establish themselves and lymphatic circulation becomes impaired. As these systems lose efficiency, toxins and metabolic waste are more likely to recirculate, hormonal signaling becomes dysregulated, and inflammatory patterns intensify across the body. Parasitic imbalance further compounds this disruption by depleting essential nutrients, weakening immune resilience, and impairing tissue repair. For this reason, meaningful recalibration cannot occur through elimination alone; sustainable restoration requires simultaneous support of digestive motility, lymphatic flow, and the intentional rebuilding of nutrient stores necessary for metabolic, endocrine, and immune stability.

The following section explores what true detoxification entails and how to prepare the body for a restorative reset that prioritizes replenishment, regulation, and long-term physiological balance rather than short-term symptom relief.

About the Author

Zaire Sabb is a clinical herbalist, traditional midwife, and educator with a deep-rooted passion for plant medicine, nourishment, and whole-body healing. Trained by the late Grand Midwife Dr. S. Ndaeyo Opio "Nana Siti" in Atlanta, Georgia, Zaire has spent years integrating traditional knowledge with contemporary herbal practice to support individuals in restoring balance and vitality. Her work centers on the belief that true healing begins by addressing the body as an interconnected system where digestion, hormones, emotional health, and spiritual wellbeing are deeply linked.

As the founder of Mystic Momma Herbals and the creator of the Roots to Remedies herbalism program, Zaire is dedicated to preserving ancestral healing traditions while making herbal knowledge practical and accessible.

Through her teaching, writing, and clinical practice, she encourages people to cultivate a deeper relationship with plants, reclaim their role in their own healing, and approach wellness as an ongoing relationship rather than a quick fix.

Zaire's work bridges education, nourishment, and ritual. In *Root & Recalibrate*, she guides readers through the foundations of clearing and restoring the body's natural balance through digestive health, detoxification, and spiritual recalibration. In *Recipe & Ritual*, she brings that process full circle by offering nourishing recipes and daily practices that help sustain vitality and deepen the relationship between food, herbs, and the body.

Originally from the United States and now living in Ghana, Zaire continues to teach, write, and develop programs that reconnect people to the wisdom of plants, the rhythms of the body, and the healing traditions carried across generations.